CBD OIL FOR PAIN RELIEF EXPLAINED!

Table of Contents

Introduction:

CBD, or Cannabidiol, is well known organic synthesis naturally created in all members of the cannabis plant family.

The health value of this astonishing phytocannabinoid was well-known to early herbal physicians and hasn't reduced one bit over the ages. Even in this age of contemporary medicine highlighting synthetic drugs of every design, the world marvels at this time-tested herbal treatment.

Today's professionals and specialists in every sphere of the medical community have commended the all-encompassing effectiveness of CBD in handling conditions of anxiety, the immune system, diet, and certain cancers.

But then, the focus of CBD benefits is its unique capability to address pain and suffering sustainably, with none of the terrible side effects connected with pharmaceutical alternatives.

Pain and the necessity for effective relief is no small matter either. According to statistics circulated by the U.S. Department of Health, more Americans suffer from depression than from diabetes, cancer, and heart disease combined. Moreover, chronic pain is the primary reason for long-term injury.

It is the diverse nature of pain and painful situations that increases the complexity of finding an effective solution. However, clinical studies are proposing that CBD could be the answer to this tough question.

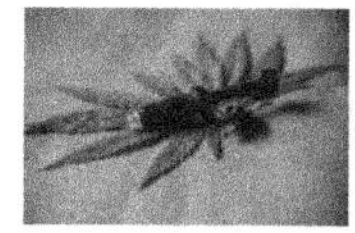

Some individuals with protracted pain use cannabidiol (CBD) oil. CBD oil may decrease pain, inflammation, and overall discomfort associated with a range of health situations. CBD oil is a product gotten from cannabis. It's a kind of cannabinoid, a chemical found indeed in marijuana and hemp plants. It doesn't cause the "high" feeling habitually associated with cannabis, which is triggered by a different type of cannabinoid called THC.

Different researches on CBD oil and pain management have shown a great deal of promise.

CBD could serve as an alternative for folks who have severe pain and depend on riskier, habit-forming medications.

Like opioids though there needs to be more study to authenticate the pain-relieving advantages of CBD oil.

CBD products aren't sanctioned by the U.S. Food and Drug Administration (FDA) for any medical situation. They aren't controlled for purity and dosage like other drugs.

CHAPTER ONE

What is CBD oil?

There are diverse levels of compounds found in the natural hemp or cannabis plant. How individuals breed the plant affects the CBD levels. Most CBD oil emanates from industrial hemp, which typically has a higher CBD content than marijuana.

Producers of CBD oil use different procedures to extract the compound. The extract is then further added to a carrier oil and named CBD oil.

CBD oil comes in numerous different strengths, and persons use it in multiple ways. It is best to have a chat on CBD oil with your doctor before using it.

CBD is genuinely known as cannabidiol oil. It is used to treat different signs though its use is somewhat contentious.

There is also some misunderstanding as to how accurately the oil affects our bodies. The oil might have health benefits, and such products that have the compound are legal in several places today.

CBD is a cannabinoid, a compound that resides in a cannabis plant.

The oil comprises CBD concentrations, and the uses vary significantly. In cannabis, the prevalent compound is delta 9 tetrahydrocannabinol or THC.

It is an active constituent found in marijuana. Marijuana has CBD and THCA, and both have different effects.

THC alters the mind when one is smoking or cooking with it. This is because it is well broken down by heat. Unlike THC, CBD isn't psychoactive.

This shows that your state of mind does not change with use. Nevertheless, substantial changes can be noted within the human body suggesting medical benefits.

Sources Of CBD Oil

Hemp is a portion of the cannabis plant, and in most cases, it is not processed. This is where a lot of the CBD is pulled out.

Marijuana and hemp come from cannabis sativa; however, there are quite different. Nowadays, marijuana farmers are breeding plants so that they could have high THC levels.

Hemp growers do not need to modify plants and are used to create the CBD oil.

For many individuals experiencing <u>chronic pain,</u> cannabidiol <u>(CBD) oil</u> has increasingly gained admiration as a logical approach to pain relief.

A compound produced in the marijuana plant, cannabidiol is at times known as an option to pain medication in the medication of common conditions like <u>arthritis</u> and <u>back pain</u>.

The usage of cannabis for pain relief dates back to ancient China, according to a <u>report</u> distributed in the journal *Cannabis and Cannabinoid Research*.

It's understood that CBD oil might help ease chronic pain in part by decreasing <u>inflammation</u>.

Furthermore, CBD oil is said to encourage sounder sleep and, in turn, treat sleep disruption usually experienced by folks with chronic pain.

It's necessary to note that several CBD oil products do not have tetrahydrocannabinol (or THC, the compound capable of offering the "high" connected with marijuana usage).

Apart from THC, cannabidiol is non-intoxicating and does not have psychoactive effects.

CHAPTER TWO

How To Make CBD Oil?

CBD oil is generally and most easily harvested from hemp and cannabis, though synthetic CBD is also accessible on the market.

There are three different procedures for obtaining CBD oil.

The beginning is the **CO2 method**, which works by pushing CO2 through the plant at high pressure and low temperature.

This extracts CBD in its cleanest form, meaning its the safest and cleanest technique of making CBD oil because it eliminates other substances, like chlorophyll, and doesn't collect any deposit.

CBD oil extracted in this way is defined as having a "cleaner taste," but is also typically the most valuable form of CBD oil.

The **ethanol method** creates CBD oil by using high-grain alcohol as a solvent for extracting. This method tends to pull more water-soluble constituents from the plant, such as chlorophyll and can end some of the useful natural oils that occur in CBD oil.

The last one is the **oil method**. This extraction technique uses a carrier oil, like olive oil, to carefully and cleanly comprise the CBD oil.

This method is rising in reputation ever since the carrier oil can add extra benefits and is free of any undesirable residues.

You should also be conscious of what your CBD is being extracted from.

If your CBD is extracted from genuine marijuana leaves rather than hemp, it can have a higher THC content (up to 33 percent) and can have psychoactive effects.

Often make sure to cross-check the THC level when buying CBD, and ask where the CBD was gotten from.

How To Take CBD Oil

If you are precisely looking to use CBD oil, first make sure that you are using quality constituents. That implies no pesticides, fungicides, or herbicides used for the duration of cultivation, no harmful contaminants, and thorough testing.

CBD comes in a range of packages which can either be swallowed or applied topically.

While consuming CBD can assist with mood-related states, like anxiety, stress, and insomnia, the topical application only relates to the topmost layers of your skin cells, so it never enters your bloodstream.

Topicals comprise **CBD instilled creams, ointments, salves, balms, patches**, or other bath and body care products.

They are superb for arthritis and injuries, but more and more skincare businesses are raving about the whole moisturizing advantages they produce on the skin, as well.

CBD could be absorbed in capsule form, oil (such as CBD infused olive oil) kind, tincture form, proper form, or by smoking or vaping.
Capsules, oil, tinctures, and vaporizing or vaping will have a very swift reaction time; somewhere between 5 to 20 minutes.

Edibles habitually take longer, somewhere from 30 minutes to two hours to take effect. Edible's effects regularly last longer, though, because of the slow way the nutrients are ingested and absorbed into the bloodstream.

Edibles comprise of gummies, sweets like lollipops and brownies, and drinks like teas and specialty sodas.
Make sure that your edibles are explicitly labeled so that they do not end up in the hands of someone who did not intend on taking CBD.

When using CBD infused olive oil, use as a salad

or veggie dressing. Heating the oil can destroy the

cannabidiols.

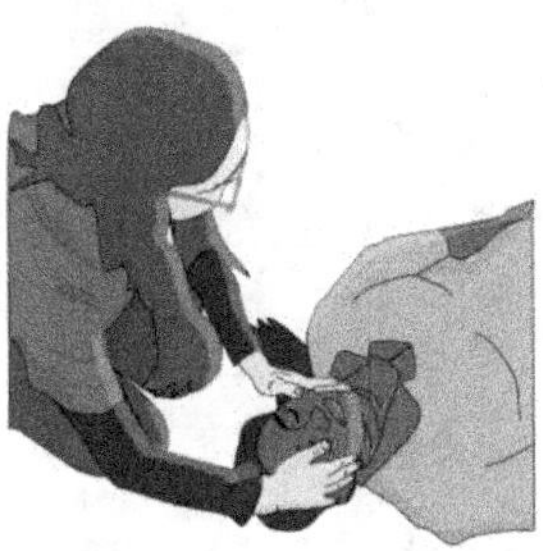

Why individuals Use CBD Oil

From the data from the Institute of Medicine of The National Academies, 110 million Americans live with chronic pain.

Along with significantly decreasing quality of life, chronic pain can increase healthcare costs and have a negative influence on productivity at work.

Common kinds of chronic pain include:

- Cancer pain
- Fibromyalgia
- <u>Headaches</u>
- <u>Irritable bowel syndrome</u> (IBS)
- <u>Low back pain</u>
- <u>Migraines</u>
- Multiple sclerosis pain
- Neuropathic pain
- <u>Osteoarthritis</u>
- Temporomandibular disorder (frequently known to as "TMJ")

Over-the-counter and prescription pain medications are always suggested in the treatment of chronic pain; however, several people lookout for alternative methods of relief (like herbs, nutritional supplements, and products like CBD oil).

Some of these persons wish to shun the side effects frequently associated with standard pain medication,

while others have grave concerns about becoming reliant on such medicines. Some protagonists suggest that CBD oil could offer a solution to opioid addiction as anxieties over opioid overdoses continue to increase.

CBD OIL VS HEMP OIL

Another major misunderstanding in the industry is a consequence of

half-truth about hemp oil (hemp seed oil) and CBD oil. **They are not at all**

the same. Comprehending the difference between the two is essential because their

appearance, chemical makeup, and users are considerably different. **Hemp oil,** also known as **hemp seed oil,** is extracted directly from hemp seeds.

The hemp seed itself comprises of up to 50% of fat in weight, which can be taken out quickly.

Hemp seeds contain a minimal amount of CBD besides; they are most frequently used for their **nutritional value as** opposed to medical use. Hemp seed oil, in contrast to CBD oil is **typically darker in appearance.**

One crucial fact to comprehend about the market is that many firms attempt to pass hemp seed oil off as a CBD product, even though

there are small traces of CBD in hemp seed oil; it just does not do justice when compared to a real CBD product.

Even though CBD oil and hemp seed oil both come from hemp, they are taking out from entirely different parts of the plant.

After industrial hemp is fermented, grown and harvested, CBD products are taking out from the flowers or buds of the plant. The oil from hemp seeds is removed before the seed ever becomes a plant. This is one of the most distinguishing factors as the oils' chemical makeups are different as their origins come from entirely different parts of the plant.

CBD always gets placed in the same category as THC (tetrahydrocannabinol),

the most well-known psychoactive compound generally associated with the marijuana plant. Even though they usually get confused with one another; they are different in chemical makeup and health benefits.

THC is hallucinogenic upon human consumption and is a prohibited substance without proper licensing in several states. It is the compound in marijuana liable for causing users to become "stoned." many products avoid this scenario absolutely as many products contain 0% THC.

CBD is a non-psychoactive compound and does not go along the same neurological routes as THC.

CBD is most commonly extracted from the hemp species, whereas THC is mostly derived from the marijuana species.

CBD products are gotten exclusively from industrial hemp never marijuana, and are free of THC which
is backed by third-party lab tests which can be seen on the label.

CHAPTER THREE

How CBD Works to EASE Pain

CBD work together with a wide range of receptors in the body and altering their function and starting physiological responses that directly affect pain and suffering.

CB1 and CB2 Endocannabinoid Receptors

CBD doesn't bind very well with the CB1 and CB2 receptors and has a negative modulating effect on their processes.

Some of these disturb pain management and help control the inflammatory response.

The majority of CBD's analgesic capability comes from its connections with several other non-cannabinoid receptors and ion channels.

Vanilloid Receptors

Well known as TRPV1 receptors, these ion channels got their name from the vanilla bean which was used to treat headaches in times past.

TRPV1 Vanilloid receptors are associated with the regulation of body temperatures, inflammation, and nociceptive pain management.

CBD binds particularly well to these ion channels and can significantly influence the experience of nociceptive pain.

Glycine Receptors

These receptors are located in the central nervous system and partake in numerous vital physiological functions comprising the control of discomfort and the inflammatory response.

CBD acts to potentiate these receptors, which affect neuropathic and nociceptive pain regulation at a spinal level.

A1A and A2A (Adenosine Receptors)

By reducing, the re-uptake of adenosine, CBD offers anti-inflammatory and anxiolytic effects.

Re-uptake is the process of enthralling neurotransmitters after their activities have been accomplished.

Adenosine controls the action of A1A and A2A receptors, which in turn add to cardiovascular function, blood pressure, myocardial oxygen depletion, and the inflammatory response.

The longer adenosine remains in the brain, the more accumulates, and this increases anti-inflammatory effects in the body.

5-HT1A Serotonin Receptor

In high adequately concentrations, CBD activates the 5-HT1A (hydroxytryptamine) serotonin receptor linked to a range of physiological and neurological processes comprising appetite, addictions, anxiety, pain perception, and nausea.

This gives analgesic and anxiolytic features for addressing a more sophisticated variety of pain and mental anguish.

On a lighter note, CBD-A, or cannabidiol acid, is the "raw" type of CBD as it endures in the bud before decarboxylation, the decline of a carbon dioxide molecule (CO_2) when cooked, smoked or vaped. CBD-A has been found to connect to these

5-HT1A serotonin receptors even better than CBD can.

The Availability of CBD Oil

As more and more states in the U.S. sanction, the use of CBD, CBD oil has become more commonly available. CBD oil is now sold in a variety of forms, as well as capsules, creams, tinctures, and under-the-tongue sprays.

Even though many firms now sell CBD oil online, and in dispensaries, the use of the oil isn't legal in most countries.

Because countries laws vary greatly when it comes to cannabis products, it's vital to check that the use of CBD oil is legal in your state.

What does CBD do for the body?

In addition to working on the brain, CBD impacts many body processes. That's because of the endocannabinoid system (ECS), which was discovered in the 1990s after scientists started examining why pot produces a high.

Though much less well-known than the cardiovascular, reproductive, and respiratory systems, the ECS is vital. "The ECS helps us to eat, sleep, relax, forget what we don't need to recall, and protect our bodies from injury," expert says.

There are added ECS receptors in the brain than there are for opioids or serotonin, including others in the intestines, liver, pancreas, ovaries, bone cells, and somewhere else.

Our bodies are known to produce endocannabinoids by the billions every day. "We often supposed the 'runner's high' was due to the release of dopamine and endorphins.

But nowadays, we recognize that the joy is also from an endocannabinoid named anandamide," its name derived from the Sanskrit word for bliss, says Joseph Maroon, MD, clinical professor and vice

chairman of neurosurgery at the University of
Pittsburgh Medical school.

We manufacture these natural chemicals all day,
but they disappear quickly since enzymes come up
to stop them. That's where CBD comes in:
By preventing these enzymes, CBD permits the
beneficial compounds to remain.
This is why Amanda johnson, 31, a career advisor
in Charleston, SC, pops a CBD gummy bear each
night before going to bed.
"I used to lie there throwing and turning as my
mind raced from work projects to whether I would
have to set the home alarm," he says.

One piece of candy with 16 milligrams (mg) of
CBD is sufficient to shut off her brain and aid
sleep.

She also asserts by the CBD oil she takes at the
height of her period, which she says quells her
devastating cramps.

CHAPTER FOUR

The Benefits Of CBD oil

Scientists are still trying to determine how CBD oil might lessen pain. Moreover, there's some proof that cannabidiol may upset the body's endocannabinoid system (a complex system of cell-to-cell communication).

Along with contributing to brain functions like memory and mood, the endocannabinoid system impacts how we experience pain.

Moreover, much of the proof for CBD's effects on pain management comes from animal-based research.

When taken orally, CBD has poor bioavailability. Topical CBD application to contained areas of pain is said to offer more reliable levels of CBD with less systemic involvement.

This research consists of a study issued in the journal *Pain* in 2017, in which scientists observed that treatment with topical CBD assists in thwarting the development of joint pain in rats with osteoarthritis.

Additional _work_, distributed in the *European Journal of Pain* in 2018, found that topical CBD gel considerably reduced joint swelling and measures of pain and inflammation in rats with arthritis.

In _research_ circulated in *Pediatric Dermatology* in 2018, scientists described three cases of topical CBD (applied as an oil, cream, and spray) use in children with a rare, blistering skin situation known as epidermolysis bullosa.
Applied by their parents, all three people conveyed faster-wound healing, some blisters, and improvement of pain.
One person was able to wean off oral opioid analgesic pain medication. There were no adverse effects stated.

CBD is valuable to human health in diverse ways. It is a regular pain reliever and has anti-inflammatory properties. Over the counter drugs are used for pain relief, and most persons prefer a more natural alternative, and this is where CBD oil comes in.

A study has shown that CBD delivers a better treatment, particularly for individuals with chronic pain.

There is also an indication that suggests that the use of CBD can be beneficial for anyone who is trying to quit smoking and dealing with drug withdrawals. In research,

it was seen that smokers who had inhalers that had CBD tend to smoke less than what was usual for them and without any further longing for cigarettes.

CBD could be a comprehensive treatment for persons with addiction disorders specifically to opioids.

CBD aids several other medical conditions, and they consist of epilepsy, LGA, Dravet syndrome, seizures, and so on.

More study is being piloted on the effects of CBD in the human body, and the results are quite encouraging.

The possibility of battling cancer and different anxiety disorders is also being looked at.

CBD oil is showing to be an excellent remedy for different kinds of conditions and ailments that affect the human body, information is power, and you will learn more about the product as you read on this ebook.

Assists as an Antitumor Promoter

If you have a tumor in your system, CBD could assist you to eradicate it. It should be taken with prescription drugs. The product lessens the growth of tumor cells in several cervical areas.

This oil is a powerful solution for the treatment of tumors in the prostate and breast areas, for instance.

2) Helps Decrease Inflammation

Ever since this oil has anti-inflammatory properties, it's one of the best agents that can assist you in creating a lot of conditions that cause pain and inflammation.

3) Helps battle Neurodegenerative Diseases

The oil can help thwart the poisonous effects of acute oxygen types and neurotransmitter glutamate in the brain. As a result, it can give security for the brain cells. The antioxidant activity of CBD is higher than vitamin E or Vitamin C.

Besides, the product can safeguard your brain cells from dangerous substances, such as toxicity from beta-amyloid. So, it could be a good cure for people with Parkinson's and Alzheimer's diseases.

4) Helps with Seizures

If you or somebody you know has seizures, CBD can assist in preventing them. According to a study comprising a lot of kids with seizures, the consistent use of this oil helped them experience a decrease in the recurrence of their seizures.

Aside from this, the kids witnessed better mood, enhanced alertness, and better sleep.

5) Decreases Anxiousness

Cannabidiol can help combat anxiety, as well. According to several studies, individuals who used this product experienced less worry while providing a public speech.

In the same way, CBD reduced anxiety initiated by THC.

6) Relieves Pain

Many researchers suggest that CBD should be used to treat persistent or chronic pain.

 Many research was done on rodents to find out if they felt relief from pain owing to the use of CBD. And the results were positive,

The rodents showed a reduction in neuropathic pain and chronic inflammation.

Benefits of Using CBD to Treat Pain

Any person suffering from acute or chronic pain should always strive for advice from a medical professional.

However, when choosing relief to the symptoms of painful situations, CBD has some distinct powers over many of the popular options out there.

- CBD is not addictive, whereas opioid-based painkillers like Vicodin and OxyContin could cause addictions and severe pain when trying to lessen doses.

- CBD has no side-effects, yet sustained use of ibuprofen has been linked with liver damage. Moreover, many OTC pain meds carry the risk of hyperalgesia, which is an amplified sensitivity to pain.

- CBD is impossible to overdose on, though it is crucial to stay within the suggested dosages of any prescription or OTC prescriptions for well-being reasons.

- CDB is desirable for long-term relief, and as of yet, there have been no reports of health risks linked with the persistent use of CBD.

For discussing conditions that can be painful for months and even years, an all-natural analgesic will place no added strain on the health.

CBD for chronic pain relief

Researchers feel that CBD relates with receptors in your brain and immune system. Receptors are tiny proteins connected to your cells that take chemical signals from different stimuli and help your cells react.

This produces anti-inflammatory and painkilling effects that assist with pain management. This means that CBD oil may benefit persons with chronic pain, such as chronic back pain.

Some scientist evaluated how good CBD works to relieve chronic pain. The assessment looked at studies piloted between the late 1980s and 2008. Based on these evaluations, researchers established that CBD was effective in overall pain management without adverse side effects.

They also stated that CBD was useful in treating insomnia associated with chronic pain.

Chronic pain

The same report considered CBD use for general chronic pain. Scientists collected the results of multiple systematic evaluations covering dozens of trials and studies.

Their research established that there is considerable evidence that cannabis is an effective treatment for chronic pain in adults.

A detailed study in the *Journal of Experimental Medicine* supports these results.

This research proposes that using CBD can decrease discomfort and swelling.

The scientist also found that subjects were not expected to build up a tolerance to the effects of CBD, so they would not need to increase their dose persistently.

They mentioned that cannabinoids, like CBD, could give helpful new treatments for individuals with chronic pain.

Regular Supplementation

Regular CBD consumption is the first step in discharging mild to severe pains in the long term. CBD edibles exist in a wide range of forms to suit any taste.

Online providers permit brownies, cookies, chewable, gummies, gel-caps, pills, drops, and tinctures.

These should be taken along with a warm meal for overall efficacy since CBD is soluble in oils and fats and not so much in the water. Effects could be slowed by the liver's enzymatic action.

Does CBD oil work for continuous pain management?

Although many folks use cannabidiol to ease pain, more scientific research is required to be sure it is safe. Understanding cannabidiol can help overcome the stigma connected with it.

Some individuals experience side effects when taking cannabidiol (CBD), and there are other factors to ponder before using CBD oil for pain.

CBD Oil Side Effects

CBD oil is regularly gotten from industrial hemp. CBD is known to be one of more than 120 compounds named cannabinoids.

Several plants consist of cannabinoids. Thus people most commonly link them to cannabis.

Not like other cannabinoids — like tetrahydrocannabinol (THC) — CBD does not produce a euphoric "high" or psychoactive effect.

This is because CBD does not alter the corresponding receptors as THC.

The human body possesses an endocannabinoid system (ECS) that collects and interprets signals from cannabinoids.

It yields some cannabinoids of its own, which are termed endocannabinoids.

The ECS assists in controlling functions such as sleep, immune-system responses, and pain.

When THC gets into the body, it produces a "high" feeling by upsetting the brain's endocannabinoid receptors. This triggers the brain's reward system, creating pleasure chemicals such as dopamine.

Does CBD make you high?

CBD is an entirely different compound from THC, and its effects are very complex.

It is not psychoactive, denoting **it does not produce a "high" or change a person's state of mind,** though it influences the body to use its endocannabinoids more efficiently.

According to one study circulated to *Neurotherapeutics*, this is for the reason that CBD itself does very little to the ECS.

In its place, it stimulates or hinders other compounds in the endocannabinoid system.

For instance, CBD stops the body from getting anandamide, a compound associated with regulating pain. Thus, increased levels of anandamide in the bloodstream might reduce the amount of anxiety an individual feels.

Cannabidiol could also lessen inflammation in the brain and nervous system, which may benefit persons experiencing pain, insomnia, and specific immune-system responses.

Other uses

In the United States, CBD oil has different legality across different states and at a federal level, yet it at present has a choice of applications and promising possibilities.

These comprise of:

- smoking cessation and drug withdrawal
- handling seizures and epilepsy
- anxiety treatment

- decreasing some of the effects of Alzheimer's, as shown by preliminary research
- antipsychotic effects on individuals with schizophrenia
- future applications in battling acne, type 1 diabetes, and cancer

Even though more study is needed to confirm some uses of CBD oil, it is shaping up as a potentially promising and useful medication.

In August 2018, the U.S. Food and Drug Administration (FDA) sanctioned one form of CBD as a treatment for people with two rare and exact kinds of epilepsy, namely Lennox-Gastaut syndrome (LGS) or Dravet syndrome (D.S.).

Dosage

The FDA does not control CBD for most conditions. As a result, dosages are presently open to explanation, and individuals should treat them with caution.

Everyone who needs to use CBD should first speak to a physician about whether it is a good plan, and how much to take.

The FDA recently approved a purified form of CBD for some types of epilepsy. If you are using this medication, be sure to follow the doctor's advice about doses.

Potential short-term side effects of using CBD oil comprise of fatigue and changes in appetite.

Most individuals tolerate CBD oil well, but there are some notable side effects.

In *Cannabis and Cannabinoid Study*, the most regular side effects include:

- tiredness
- diarrhea
- changes in appetite
- weight gain or weight loss

In addition, using CBD oil with other medications could make those medications more or less effective.

The experts also state that scientists have yet to study some aspects of CBD, such as its long-term effects on hormones. Further long-term studies will be beneficial in defining any side effects CBD has on the body over time.

CBD and other cannabinoids might also put the consumer at risk for lung problems.

One study also revealed that cannabinoids' anti-inflammatory effect might lessen inflammation too much.

A large decline in inflammation could reduce the lungs' defense system, increasing the possibility of infection.

Other considerations

Almost all study on CBD oil and pain emanates from adult trials. Experts do not endorse CBD oil for use in children, as there is little research on the effects of CBD oil on a child's developing brain.

Folks should turn to their doctor if they feel a child needs to use CBD oil for seizures.

CBD oil is also not suggested during pregnancy or while breastfeeding.

CHAPTER FIVE

What sorts of Pain Can Cannabidiol (CBD) Treat?

Pain, when used in a general term, is more enormous than the Pacific Ocean. Using CBD to handle pain can be effective only under the pretense that the type of pain is well-understood and appropriately diagnosed.

Many of us have crossed paths with the intense, penetrating, cuss-worthy persona of severe pain: an elbow touches the edge of the table or a pinky toe that has found the bed frame yet again at 4 a.m.

Other kinds of pain produce less shock value but are no less odious in nature.

For the sake of this eBook, I'll basically go into the types of pain that CBD has shown to treat effectively: neuropathic and inflammatory pain.

Cannabis has been utilized for relief for thousands of years and CBD, one of the active compounds in the cannabis plant species has been particularly valued.

In olden Chinese texts dating back to 2900 B.C., cannabis is termed as a form of relief from particular joint discomfort.

The plant was also employed in combination with wine before some methods. And in India, about 1000 B.C., cannabis was treasured as an overall health supporter.

Though many compounds of the cannabis plant were used in ancient health approaches, comprising the psychoactive compound THC, we know from more modern studies that CBD is a calming powerhouse on its own. Pain relief is one of the most reputable CBD oil advantages, and for a good reason, as the compound works to overpower certain processes and signals in the brain to offer relief

That's why many contemplate using CBD oil. With many in the hunt for relief from occasional discomfort, it's about time we look to Cbd oil for soothing relief.

Types of Pain

Basically, the pain has been categorized into two classes, neuropathic pain, and nociceptive pain.

These are both entirely different in their basic biological mechanism and therefore need very different treatments to address properly.

Nociceptive Pain

When nerve fibers are stimulated as a result of a chemical, mechanical or inflammatory stimulus, nociceptive pain is experienced as an alert response to the brain.

Nociceptive pain is the flavor behind the stubbed toe, the insect bite, and inflammatory conditions, as well as some hidden pain from old injuries.

Neuropathic pain

This is the type of pain sustained or produced in the nervous system and comprises such hard to treat conditions like multiple sclerosis, diabetes, cancer, and other nervous conditions.

Conventional pain treatment has been found less effective against neuropathic pain.

Other Types of Pain

In addition to Neuropathic and Nociceptive pain, there are a few other forms of pain that don't suitably fit into either category.

Fibromyalgia and the painful symptoms connected with this condition, like migraine headaches, can cause diverse painful responses that are particularly difficult to treat. Occasionally,
the combination of nociceptive and neuropathic pain is complemented by extreme depression or fear, and treatment for these pains needs the application of antidepressants to address it correctly.

How CBD Works for Pain

CBD hampers glutamate release and other inflammatory agents, which makes it 'neuroprotective' and outstanding at dulling the prickling, tingling and burning sensations that neuropathic pain is known for. CBD oil could be used as a supplement to support in managing neuropathic pain, alongside other natural supplements such as magnesium glycinate.

Pain due to inflammation is not as simply categorized as other types of pain, generally because its origins of pain vary, and so does the experience.

On the optimistic side, CBD is decent at calming inflammation, no matter what the root cause is.

The anti-inflammatory mechanism of cannabidiol is exclusive to cannabis. It doesn't work like other anti-inflammatory drugs by hindering COX-1 and COX-2 receptors, which means you don't run the risk of developing gastrointestinal ulcers or heart attacks, hurrah!

Several studies have shown that cannabinoids (CBD is up to twenty times more powerful anti-inflammatory agents when equated to NSAIDs (eg. Ibuprofen).

When taken on a regular basis alongside other natural anti-inflammatory supplements (e.g., curcumin, Omega-3), CBD can offer systemic relief of inflammation.

Regularly taken three times per day, dosing at each interval hinge on your unique needs. Normally, patients start with 0.5 mg per dose and increase until maximum relief.

Cannabidiol can be an effective, non-psychotropic substitute to THC when used properly. Nevertheless, we are still in the infancy stage of integrating CBD into health and medicine,
so it is essential to check in your physician when anticipating the use of CBD to treat pain.

It's imperative to remember that CBD oil, like other nutraceuticals, can work together with medications.

The takeaway? CBD is very efficient in treating all types of pain—for that reason, it's vital to comprehend your pain: does it deteriorate with the weather, cause swelling, or is it persistent and stabbing? If you feel that you experience inflammatory or neuropathic pain, talk to your doctor. CBD supplementation could be right for you.

Can CBD oil be used for pain-Relieving?

Presently, the answer is yes. CBD is an alternative for many pain patients to help relieve their symptoms, owing to its antioxidant properties.

'CBD oil is one of the most useful supplements to become obtainable in a long time,' says Dr. Johnson.

'It is exceedingly antioxidant so has anti-inflammatory effects on joints, to improve pain and stiffness. CBD also has an analgesic effect of lessening pain perception in the brain.'

Cannabidiol (CBD) is now used internationally for a variety of medical conditions, including pain relief.

This is following several studies showing that some of the best CBD oils can have a particularly positive bearing on pain management.

It's vital to note that CBD oil isn't yet fully approved by the U.S. Food and Drug Administration for any medical condition, which means that the products discussed and statements made in this ebook have been partially assessed by the FDA and are not intended to make a diagnosis, treat, cure or avert any disease.

Even with the partial FDA's review, CBD has been getting a substantial amount of attention, even being featured on some of the top news networks who have all applauded its achievements.

For illustration, Charlotte's Web, at present categorized as one of the worlds best CBD Oil manufacturers, has been presented numerous times in the media on sites such as CNN, The Wall Street Journal, BBC and even in health magazines like Men's Health.

They are also a publicly-traded company.

"CBD is known as one of the most captivating additives or isolate we have known in recent years.

Whereas most pharmaceutical medications emphasis on the symptoms or one enzyme or channel of the human body, CBD aids in helping a system to function more efficiently. The endocannabinoid system."

CBD Oil for Relief

CBD oil works to relieve discomfort in astonishing ways. In fact, scientists are finding out that the endocannabinoid system relates to many points with our main bodily control systems.

This biological system is working in support of general comfort, and cannabinoids that respond to receptors in the system are able to work to lessen discomfort.

Numerous studies have investigated the positive effects of cannabis compounds, including both THC and CBD.

We have learned from this study that CBD oil is able to ease many types of discomfort by interacting with receptors in our brains.

One area of relief always connected with CBD oil is occasional joint discomfort. Though more research needs to be piloted, some research shows that it may be a valuable approach to supporting overall joint comfort.

How quickly can I anticipate to see results?

How quickly CBD oil works rest on the delivery method, you choose.

'Capsules normally have a slow action, and can take from 23 minutes to an hour to produce the anticipated outcome,' says Dr. James.

In additional, 'oral sprays and liquid drips of CBD, which could be held in the mouth to increase absorption directly into the circulation, work more quickly – you might notice an effect within just a few minutes.'

The effects of CBD typically last for around three to five hours. 'After this,' the expert says, 'the dose will have fallen below levels that produce obvious advantages.'

☐**Do not ingest CBD if you are pregnant or breastfeeding. If you are on any prescriptions, check for interactions with your doctor.**

CHAPTER SIX

How to Utilize CBD Oil for Pain — Dosage Information

There are a few means that you can use CBD oil for pain. This is a breakdown of what's at present accessible and can be applied orally or topically for pain relief:

- **Oils:** The most efficient CBD oils are full-spectrum, which means that they contain all compounds found naturally in the plant, comprising the cannabinoids (with trace amounts of THC), terpenes and basic oils. You could put CBD oils in a bottle with a dropper. This permits you to ingest the oil by placing it under your tongue, letting it sit for about 16 seconds and then swallowing it.

- **Tinctures:** Tinctures are another common way to use CBD, likely because you can simply gauge precisely how much cannabidiol you are ingesting, like CBD oil. A tincture is typically gotten with alcohol or another solvent. With a tincture, you could use a dropper and place the drops under your tongue. At times, companies will use carrier oils, native flavors, or fatty oils in their tinctures.

- **Capsules:** CBD capsules can be applied orally with water. You'll be able to obtain CBD capsules in a variety of doses, normally in amounts of 10–50 milligrams.

  Capsules could be taken once to three times daily, dependent on the severity of discomfort.

- **Powder:** CBD powder can be combined with smoothies, juices, water, or any kind of beverage. Check the label for dosage instructions.

- **Topical solution:** Topical salves, lotions, and gels comprising CBD are obtainable and can be applied appropriately to areas of pain, like the lower back, neck, knees, hands, and feet. See the product label for directions and potency.

How much CBD oil must you use for pain?

There is no approved serving size for CBD oil since everyone reacts in a different way to cannabinoids.

In order to know the right CBD oil dosage to lessen your pain, you'll want to take a few things into the reckoning.

- **What are your goals?** In order to ascertain the right CBD oil dosage for you, you'll require to define your health goals. If you are looking for pain relief, state what type of pain you are hoping to reduce.

  This will let you monitor the effectiveness of your initial CBD dose and decide whether or not it's doing the job.

- **What is your severity of pain?** Your CBD dosage will rest on your condition, so you (in conjunction with your healthcare expert) will need to classify your personal needs as low, medium, high, or very high.

  - Low — start with a 6–11-milligram dose
  - Medium — start with an 11–21-milligram dose
  - High or very high — begin with a 22–41-milligram dose

- **Is my starting dosage working?** As soon as you and your healthcare expert have identified your exact goals stabilized your situation, you'll commence with an initial CBD dosage.

- It's more satisfying to start with lower doses and work your way up. Why? Since everyone has a different sensitivity to cannabis compounds.

Some persons only need a very small amount to notice the beneficial effects, while others might need higher doses.

- Start on the lower end of your suggested dosage range and take that amount regularly for 3–7 days.

    Keep going back to your primary goals and appraise whether this starting dose is improving your symptoms.

- Is it working? Great! Stick with this dose, which could be taken 1–3 times daily or according to directions and your healthcare specialist.

    - Don't notice any progresses yet? Then check with your healthcare specialist to see if you can increase your dose by 6 milligrams and stick with this new amount for another 3–7 days.

How prolonged does it take CBD oil to work for pain relief? It's normally suggested that you use CBD oil about one hour before desired benefits. Typically, you'll notice the positive effects in 32–62 minutes.

The gains of CBD oil for pain will last about 5–7 hours, dependent on the dosage. If you have other needs, then you might benefit from taking a dose every five hours or so.

CBD Oil Precautions

The current research recommends that CBD usage has few and in general mild side effects, and a "tolerance" for CBD does not appear to occur. Whenever you are looking at CBD vs. THC, it's THC that has the mind-altering consequences that make you appear "high." CBD does not have intoxicating consequences.

Presently, there are a lot of CBD products in the marketplace, so you need to shop carefully. Only use CBD oil products that are examined for contaminants and show CBD vs. THC levels.

Look for a product that has got a COA, or certificate of analysis, which make sure that it has been tested and met lab standards.

It's also highly suggested that you go with an organic CBD oil. The hemp plant is a "bio-accumulator," which implies that it's capable of absorbing toxic elements from the soil, water, and air quicker than the rate they're lost.

So going natural for all of your CBD products will safeguard that you aren't also ingesting toxic pesticides and other chemicals.

Chronic Pain By the Numbers

Chronic pain is more than a typical injury, pulled muscle, or troublesome headache. By description and various diagnosis principles, the pain reaches the "chronic" level when it has persisted endlessly for 12 weeks or more.

Rather than standard pain signals that let us know there's an injury, chronic pain is persistent, and relief is problematic to come by.

It could be created by an injury or primary illness, or it causes may be problematic to difficult to identify.

Regrettably, chronic pain doesn't stand alone. It's often complemented by:

- Tiredness
- Restiveness
- Inability to sleep
- Reduced appetite
- Noticeable mood swings and changes
- Restricted movement
- Reduced strength
- Depression
- Nervousness
- And more

Physicians are regularly hesitant to diagnose chronic pain pending all other treatable conditions have been ruled out.

Because of this, diagnosis and the evolution of a formal treatment plan can take months or even years.

Getting a diagnosis can also be costly. Many times, extensive tests are required to rule out all likely "definitive" answers, comprising MRI, CT scans, blood tests, and more.

Each of these comes with a price – comprising the real cost of the test, time out of work, and more. The weight of diagnosing chronic pain disorders is great.

During the waiting period, physicians might give different treatment options and pain management medications, going from injections to opioids and more; which we will cover soon.

This is particularly frustrating for the individual suffering pain and their loved ones – especially when something simple, like suggesting the patient use CBD oil, could solve the problem or at least offer relief. Since this is not an FDA approved option, yet, this isn't an option

Nowadays, chronic pain affects more than 110 million Americans; that's more than diabetes, heart conditions, and cancer put together.

It is far from unique, and the need for an antidote and the need for respite have never been more vital.

THE COST OF CHRONIC PAIN:

The total yearly incremental cost of health care coming from pain ranges from **$565 billion to $638 billion** in the U.S.

This comprises medical costs, lost wages, and lost productivity in the workplace.

OTHER FAST FACTS

NUMEROUS AMERICAN ADULTS FEEL PAIN FROM A LACK OF SLEEP A FEW NIGHTS A WEEK OR MORE OWING TO CHRONIC PAIN

PEOPLE GRIEFING FROM PAIN – SUCH AS BACK PAIN – ARE FREQUENTLY FOUND TO BE IN WORSE PHYSICAL SHAPE, AND MENTAL HEALTH THAN THOSE WHO DO NOT

THE MOST USUALLY REPORTED KINDS OF CHRONIC PAIN COMPRISE:

THE ALTERNATIVE YOU'VE BEEN LOOKING FOR MIRACLE RELIEF?

If customary medications and narcotics fall short for chronic pain relief, what are victims to do?

This is where the benefits of CBD oil not only enter the fray but then steal the show.

Emerging studies have begun to prove the power of CBD to get rid of the pain – even modest to severe pain.

A thrilling advance in 2018 (in the form of clinical trials) proven the efficiency of non-intoxicating cannabinoid compounds like CBD in relating directly with neural pathways that control pain, offering a gifted alternative course of treatment for patients looking for a non-narcotic treatment plan or for patients for whom old treatments have fallen short.

This year, investigators found that CBD is effective in regulating inflammation and pain (which habitually stem from issues with the immune system) without generating an analgesic tolerance that could lead to difficulty and/or withdrawal symptoms at the conclusion of treatment.

Some lab examinations test the use of CBD for definite conditions like multiple sclerosis (M.S.). For example, researchers in 2017 finished a double-blind, placebo-controlled study which concluded that CBD could aid treating neuropathic pain that most patients label "debilitating," and another study the same year delivered comparable results in a CBD-based drug trial for patients with M.S.

A study that took place in 2018 concluded that CBD is, in fact, efficient for therapeutic neuropathic pain relief.

There are few of the numerous studies that have been completed and are directing patients toward something promising, something better.
The positive effects of CBD are truly spectacular, and we're just starting to discover the opportunity for more. Who remembered something as easy as a plant compound could deliver so much.

HOW DOES CBD OIL REDUCE PAIN?

As additional cannabinoid receptors were revealed, the complete endocannabinoid system in human bodies, one intended to relate with and parallel other systems in the body that manage pain, came to light.

Whenever the endocannabinoid system is able to work correctly, the body is more expected to respond well to pain, even when traditional treatments fall short.

The endocannabinoid system contains several receptors (largely CB1 and CB2 receptors) that react to cannabinoids, releasing enzymes all through the central nervous system, brain and rest of the body that stimulate balance decrease the effects of injurious chemicals that build up in the body, lessen inflammation – a foremost professional in persistent pain, arthritis pain – and more.

That's why, for some time, medical cannabis has been a top choice for treating chronic pain.

The body is planned to respond to this natural substance, eradicating negative stressors throughout it. In other words, CBD oil – along with other cannabinoids – work, even when other drugs, morphine incorporated, fall short because our bodies have a system that is designed to use them to their fullest extent.

HOW TO DEFINE YOUR CBD DOSAGE AND ROUTINE FOR PAIN RELIEF

Won over still?

If not, that's okay – be certain to speak to your medical provider about whether CBD may be most desirable for you.

If you are hell-bent on giving it a try, discovering the regimen and amount of CBD that's right concerning your definite needs is mission-critical.

Like traditional pain treatment strategies, you may require a daily maintenance schedule, along with an option for when a flare does happen.

For regular maintenance, you have to learn how to take CBD oil. You can pick whichever product that feels correct for you; a tincture that dissolves under the tongue, oil, capsules, or more.

Each of these ingested forms of CBD permits the compound to enter your body certainly, though the time before desired relief sets in may differ and may be longer when ingested in these forms.

Several users report starting with a 6-11 mg CBD dose every day, whereas others find relief with a standard 26 mg per day regimen. As with other drugs, I am starting slowly and slowly improving is often best.

If no change is felt at this level, increase by another 6-11 mg of CBD till relief is felt.

Beginning at a higher dose, the first time is not always required or desirable; start with a lower dose until you find your sweet spot.

Though, different conditions may necessitate different, or even higher doses.

It's significant to note that patients looking for pain in a precise area of the body, on the skin or connecting to a muscle may want to explore a topical lotion, rather than CBD in an ingestible form.

What about a flare-up?

No drug can totally eradicate the chance of a pain flare-up since oftentimes; these flares are caused by exterior situations or variables – the weather, too much activity, heat, stress, or something else.

When this happens, many victims find relief in a vaporized or inhaled version of CBD oil. This permits for a more rapid effect, instead of the delayed onset connected with ingestible forms of CBD oil, though, the effects are habitually more short term. Just something to keep in mind.

Another option is depending on a CBD oil tincture when a pain flare arises. CBD tinctures (in a range of CBD oil dosages) can be dropped under the tongue and held for 32 to 63 seconds before swallowing. In this method, CBD starts to take effect in 12-22 minutes, with a heightened effect in 62 minutes. CBD oil tinctures can be flavored in numerous flavors, some more needed than others. Finding the one that's right for your desires might take some experimentation. They also come in a variety of energies.

Other kinds of ingesting edibles comprise CBD capsules, CBD isolate, oil and CBD cannabutter baked into baked goods and more. The choices are approximately endless and appropriate for a variety of medical conditions, and you can vary the serving size for your needs.

Check out a CBD dosage calculator to decide the right dose of CBD to start with for your body weight and other factors. Finding the proper dosage is vital!

CHAPTER SEVEN

DOES CBD OIL HAVE SIDE EFFECTS?

Good,you have a lot in mind, and you're waiting to start. But, if traditional pain relief treatment options have numerous side effects, CBD has to as well…right?

The answer might interest you.

 CBD oil side effects do exist… But these effects are seldom reported. They include:

- **Tiredness.**
- **Stomach effects comprising diarrhea.**
- **Appetite alteration.**
- **Weight gain or loss.**

The most satisfying part? CBD's impacts are not life-threatening, and overdosing is virtually impossible. It is one of the only substances described to have no serious side effects by the World Health Organization.

When equated with the major – sometimes life-threatening – risks of traditional pain management, it's perfect that CBD is a nice-looking alternative, worth trying.

Furthermore, using CBD oil with other medications may make those medications more or less efficient.

The appraisal also notes that scientists have yet to study some aspects of CBD, such as its long-term effects on hormones.
Further long-term studies will be useful in shaping any side effects CBD has on the body over time.
Persons who are considering using CBD oil should converse with their doctors.
Doctors will want to observe the person for any changes and make adjustments as a result.

The patient info leaflet for most cbd oil cautions that there is a threat of liver damage, lethargy, and probably depression and thoughts of suicide, but these are true of other treatments for epilepsy, too.

CBD and other cannabinoids might also put the consumer at danger for lung problems.

Further study in *Frontiers in Pharmacology*, recommended cannabinoids' anti-inflammatory effect may decrease inflammation too much.

A huge reduction in inflammation could lessen the lungs' defense system, increasing the danger of infection

HOW TO DISCOVER THE Correct CBD FOR YOUR PAIN MANAGEMENT NEEDS?

As you read through the report presented above, you might have recognized that CBD does have many variables.

Some of these are connected to the fact that the science around CBD oil is fairly "new," all things considered, others relate to the fact that so many choices and forms are obtainable for those looking into CBD products.

Because the compound is not yet controlled by any federal agencies, be careful, targeted research is totally essential.

The science is in; the research is ongoing: CBD may offer a needed option to conventional pain management. Relief could be more possible than ever.

As you dive in, take the time to explore numerous forms of CBD, to test what works for you, and to create your own regimen for getting rid of the pain. Traditional pain relief opportunities are not your only choices; side effect free options – like pure CBD – do exist.

How to Use CBD for Pain Management

Possibly the most widespread use for CBD is for pain management. The truth is that pain will affect every person at some point in his or her life, and it's reassuring to know that there is a natural remedy that can help. The use of a natural remedy is particularly essential for those suffering from neuropathic pain and chronic pain – or pain that lasts for more than a few months.

Does chronic pain affect more than 20 million people all over the world every year – and the worst part? It can't be cured.

Nevertheless, it can be handled. The paradox is that in the United States, the most popular medical treatments are nerve blocks, steroids, and narcotics (opioids) – many of which carry the substantial prospect of side effects and obsession. Even over the counter non-steroidal anti-inflammatory medicines (NSAIDs) such as Aspirin and ibuprofen are risky when used frequently – hospitalizing over 170,000 folks each year and killing approximately 20,000. Furthermore, risky narcotics and NSAIDs are not your only choice for pain alleviation!

Moreover, to physical therapy and self-care, you can integrate CBD oil into your treatment regimen for natural, plant-based pain relief. CBD is basically different than most recommended painkillers, as it's not addictive, non-toxic, and has very slight (if any unspecified) side effects.

Whether the lingering pain is in your back, neck, hands, feet, or somewhere else – CBD oil can ease it! In order to comprehend how CBD helps relief pain relief, we turn to a series of medical studies that have been piloted over the past eleven years. These studies appraised CBD's medical efficacy in treating those who suffer from numerous types of pain. We will address the results below.

Study Results:

A 2017 research looked at the effects of cannabinoids in treating the devastating pain experienced by 55-75% of multiple sclerosis (M.S.) patients. The double-blind placebo-controlled research proven that ***"cannabinoids comprising the cannabidiol (CBD)/THC buccal spray are effective in treating neuropathic pain in M.S."***

Suggested CBD Regimen for Pain Management

When formulating a CBD schedule for a particular disease or illness (like chronic or neurological pain), it's vital to comprehend that CBD should be used frequently for maximum relief.

Meaning it should be used as a preemptive first – it can also be used to manage acute flare-ups, though the preventative maintenance is most significant! Think about it like any other dietary supplement; you desire to institute a baseline concentration in your system.

Everyday Maintenance

In order to manage pain, we recommend swallowing CBD oil daily in the kind of Tinctures or Gel Capsules.

The constituents in the two products are the same; the only change between the two is the form factor and dosage – pills vs. sublingual tinctures. We propose those suffering from any kind of pain start with 6-11mg per day of CBD. If relief is not observed at this dosage, we recommend taking 6-11mg until the desired effects are accomplished.

You'll see that the Gel Capsules are pre-filled and contain 28mg of CBD per pill – there is no harm in starting at 28mg CBD every day as you cannot overdose on CBD nor are there any grave side effects.

These ingestible products provide continuous relief for numerous hours – many persons find they offer relief for the whole day!

The one thing to keep in mind with ingestible CBD products is the slowed onset time – it can take up to 110 minutes for the full effects of the tinctures or capsules to be felt.

For pain located in the skin, bones, muscle, ligaments, tendons, or myofascial tissue, we also suggest supplementing with a topical salve like the Deep Rub. This extra strength salve pierces deep beneath the skin layer to lessen inflammation and pain. Relief can be felt within 20 minutes and lasts several hours. Simply re-apply as needed.

Handling Acute Flare-Ups

Furthermore, the daily pain management program stated above, many individuals find they still need a safe way to accomplish acute flare-ups.

Whether it's triggered by a recent injury, cold weather, or complete aggravation – we recommend vaporizing CBD isolate to fight these acute pain flare-ups.

The advantage of vaporizing or dabbing CBD isolate is that the relief can be felt almost promptly. CBD isolate is 99% pure CBD and offers a wave of relief that can be felt all through the whole body.

You can also take more CBD in the form of tinctures or pills to battle these flare-ups, just keep in mind that the onset time will be considerably longer than sublimating. CBD topical salves can also be used to accomplish acute pain flare-ups.

If you are ready to give it a try, finding the regimen and amount of CBD that's right for your specific needs is mission-critical.

Like traditional pain treatment plans, you may need a daily maintenance schedule, along with an option for when a flare does occur.

It's imperative to note that patients looking for pain in a particular area of the body, on the skin or connecting to a muscle may want to investigate a topical lotion, rather than CBD in an ingestible form.

What about a flare-up?
No drug can totally eliminate the chance of a pain flare-up since oftentimes; these flares are caused by external conditions or variables – the weather, too much activity, heat, stress, or something else.

When this happens, many sufferers find relief in a vaporized or inhaled version of CBD. This allows for a more immediate effect, instead of the delayed onset linked with ingestible forms of CBD, but, the effects are habitually more short term. Just something to keep in mind.

Another option is depending on a CBD tincture when a pain flare occurs. CBD tinctures (in a range of CBD oil dosages) can be dropped under the tongue and held for 35 to 65 seconds before swallowing.

In this method, CBD commences taking effect in 15-25 minutes, with a keen effect in 63 minutes.

CBD oil tinctures can be spice up in various flavors; some are more alluring than others. Discovering the one that's right for your needs may take some research.

They also appear in a range of strengths.

Other means of eating edibles comprise of CBD capsules, CBD isolate, oil and CBD cannabutter baked into baked goods and more.

The choices are approximately endless and appropriate for a variety of medical conditions, and you can vary the serving size for your needs.

Check out a CBD dosage calculator to regulate the right dose of CBD to start with for your body weight and other factors. Finding the proper dosage is critical!

A Quick Note About CBD & Drug Testing

If drug testing is a section of the provisions of your employment, you might be disturbed about the potential of CBD to prompt you to test positive for THC.

This isn't an unfounded interest -- though, there isn't precisely a cut-and-dry way to answer it.

Much of the details we have about CBD is circumstantial, and its potential impact on drug testing is no exemption.

There are some few peer-reviewed studies on the subject, but there seems to be a small risk of a false positive for some users.

Shunning CBD products comprising traces of THC can lessen your risk of a false positive, but that may not eradicate the risk completely.

If you are worried about passing a drug test, you should ponder this potential risk when deciding whether CBD is right for you.

CBD Oil Side Effects and Precautions

The contemporary research infers that CBD usage has few and usually mild side effects, and a "tolerance" for CBD does not appear to happen. While you are looking at CBD vs. THC, it's THC that has the mind-altering effects that make you appear "high." CBD does not have intoxicating effects.

What to look out for in a quality CBD oil

Pick products made with American hemp

Even though CBD oils aren't controlled by the FDA, buying products stateside from one of the nine states where recreational and medical cannabis use is lawful will possible result in a higher-quality product than buying one made with hemp-derived CBD oil bring in from abroad, says Martin Jay, director of Project CBD, a nonprofit that encourages medical investigation into CBD.

Go for "full-spectrum" or "broad-spectrum"

These expressions mean that all or most of the constituents that can be extracted from the hemp plant are concentrated in the oil. The broader the range of components involved, versus just CBD, the greater the potential medicinal benefit of the product, says Jay.

Note the quantity of CBD and THC per dose

There's no fixed amount that's suitable for everyone, but the ratio of CBD to THC will indicate how psychoactive the product is and if it's legal in your state. The more CBD equated with THC, the less of a high, and vice versa.

 "Managing psych activity is key to popular cannabis therapy," says Jay. "Values should be made clear on the label and lab-certified, so folks know what's helping them and what's not."

Conclusion:

CBD oil has a potent component in which several kinds of research claim it can help with everything from chronic pain relief to treating cancer.

Furthermore, CBD oil does show a lot of prospect for pain relief. Anecdotal sign advocates that it can be used to help manage chronic pain in numerous cases.

CBD oil is exceptionally encouraging due to the shortage of intoxicating effects and a sustainable lower potential for side effects than several other pain medications.

Individuals should discuss CBD oil with their doctor if they are considering using it for the first time.

www.ingramcontent.com/pod-product-compliance
Lightning Source LLC
Chambersburg PA
CBHW050652250726
48662CB00002B/625